LOW-POTASSIUM MEALS FOR KIDNEY HEALTH

Delicious and Nutritious Recipes to Support Kidney Function

Dr Lily Morgan

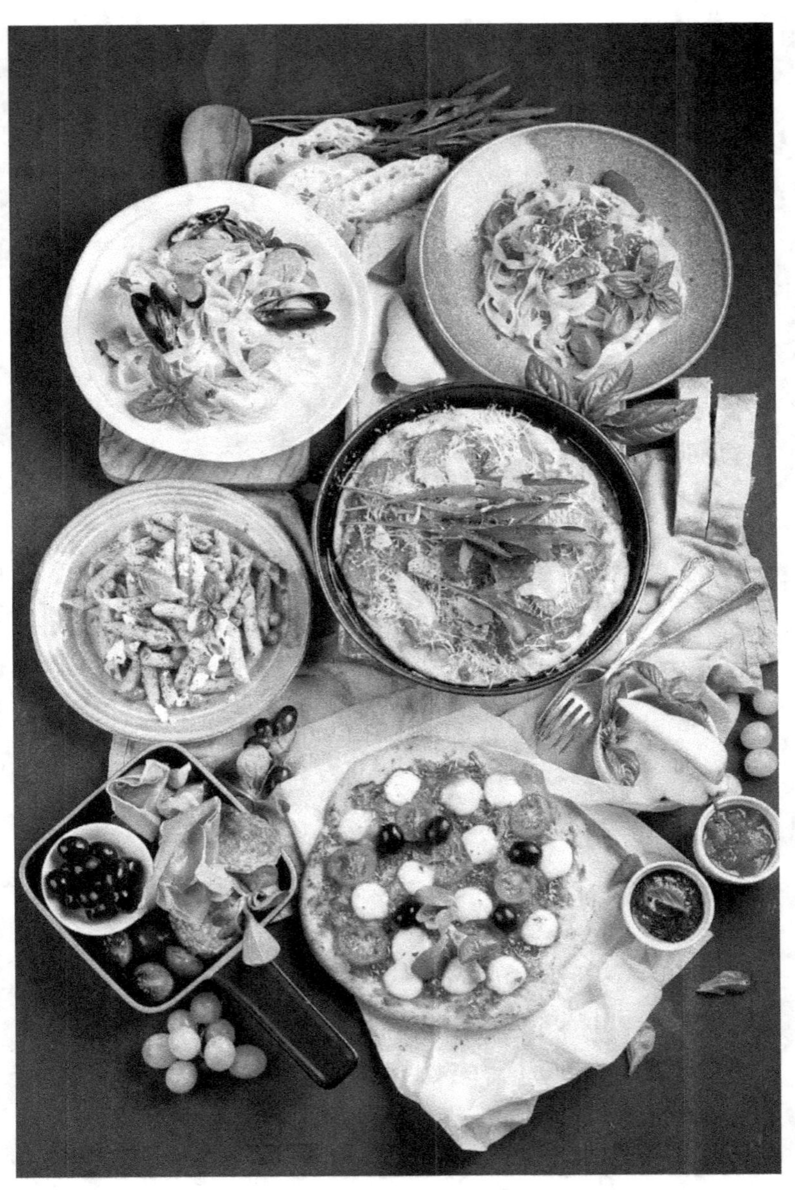

TABLE OF CONTENTS

Chapter 3: Lunch Recipes 36

Chapter 6: Desserts 80

INTRODUCTION

The kidneys, those remarkable bean-shaped organs nestled deep within our abdomen, are the unsung heroes of our body's filtration system. While they may not grab headlines like the heart or brain, their role in maintaining our overall health cannot be understated. These fist-sized powerhouses work tirelessly to remove waste and excess fluids from our blood, regulate blood pressure, and produce essential hormones. Understanding kidney health is a fundamental step towards safeguarding our well-being.

Importance of a Low-Potassium Diet:

One crucial aspect of maintaining kidney health is monitoring our potassium intake. Potassium, a vital mineral found in many foods, plays a pivotal role in nerve function, muscle contractions, and maintaining a steady heartbeat. However, for individuals with compromised kidney function, too much potassium in the bloodstream can be a serious concern. High levels of potassium can disrupt the delicate balance of electrolytes in the body, leading to irregular heart rhythms and other health complications. This is where a low-potassium diet steps in as a key ally. By carefully selecting and preparing foods, individuals with kidney issues can better control their potassium intake, helping to manage their condition effectively.

Tips for Managing Potassium Intake:

Managing potassium intake doesn't have to be an overwhelming task; it's all about making informed choices. Here are some practical tips to keep potassium levels in check:

1. **Be Mindful of High-Potassium Foods:** Knowing which foods are potassium-rich is the first step. Common culprits include bananas, oranges, potatoes, and spinach. While these are nutritious, moderation is key.

2. **Cooking Methods Matter:** Certain cooking techniques can leach potassium from foods. For

instance, soaking vegetables in water before cooking can reduce their potassium content.

3. **Portion Control:** Controlling portion sizes is an effective strategy. Smaller servings of high-potassium foods can help limit potassium intake.

4. **Read Labels:** When shopping for packaged foods, scrutinize labels for potassium content. Some processed foods may contain hidden sources of potassium.

5. **Consult a Dietitian:** For those with specific dietary restrictions due to kidney issues, seeking guidance from a registered dietitian or nutritionist is invaluable. They can tailor meal plans to individual needs.

6. **Stay Hydrated**: Drinking enough water helps dilute potassium in the body, so staying adequately hydrated is essential.

In summary, understanding kidney health and the significance of a low-potassium diet is pivotal for individuals aiming to protect and improve their overall well-being. By following these tips for managing potassium intake, one can navigate the path to kidney health with confidence and control.

Chapter 1: 30-Day Meal Plan

Week 1:

Day 1:

- Breakfast: Low-Potassium Oatmeal with Berries
- Lunch: Chicken and Vegetable Stir-Fry
- Dinner: Grilled Chicken Breast with Lemon
- Snacks: Veggie Sticks with Hummus
- Dessert: Berry Parfait with Whipped Cream

Day 2:

- Breakfast: Scrambled Egg Whites with Spinach
- Lunch: Tuna Salad with Low-Potassium Ingredients
- Dinner: Baked Cod with Herbed Potatoes
- Snacks: Low-Potassium Salsa and Chips
- Dessert: Apple Crisp (in moderation)

Day 3:

- Breakfast: Greek Yogurt Parfait with Nuts
- Lunch: Quinoa and Chickpea Salad
- Dinner: Quinoa-Stuffed Bell Peppers

- Snacks: Cottage Cheese Dip with Veggies
- Dessert: Chocolate Avocado Mousse

Day 4:

- Breakfast: Banana-Free Smoothie
- Lunch: Turkey Wrap with Hummus
- Dinner: Beef and Broccoli Stir-Fry
- Snacks: Guacamole with Cucumber Slices
- Dessert: Poached Pears

Day 5:

- Breakfast: Quinoa Breakfast Bowl
- Lunch: Baked Salmon with Herbs
- Dinner: Eggplant Parmesan
- Snacks: Roasted Chickpeas
- Dessert: Rice Pudding (in moderation)

Day 6:

- Breakfast: Avocado Toast with Low-Potassium Toppings
- Lunch: Spinach and Lentil Soup
- Dinner: Teriyaki Salmon

- Snacks: Mixed Nuts (in moderation)
- Dessert: Angel Food Cake with Berries

Day 7:

- Breakfast: Cereal Alternatives
- Lunch: Low-Potassium Pasta Salad
- Dinner: Creamy Mushroom Risotto
- Snacks: Fruit Sorbet
- Dessert: Lemon Sorbet

Week 2:

Day 8:

- Breakfast: Sweet Potato Hash Browns
- Lunch: Lentil and Vegetable Curry
- Dinner: Lemon Herb Shrimp
- Snacks: Rice Cakes with Toppings
- Dessert: Pumpkin Pie (in moderation)

Day 9:

- Breakfast: Low-Potassium Pancakes
- Lunch: Greek Salad with Feta
- Dinner: Stuffed Cabbage Rolls

- Snacks: Baked Sweet Potato Fries
- Dessert: Chia Seed Chocolate Pudding

Day 10:

- Breakfast: Breakfast Burrito with Kidney-Friendly Ingredients
- Lunch: Roasted Veggie and Couscous Bowl
- Dinner: Pork Tenderloin with Apple Sauce
- Snacks: Edamame
- Dessert: Low-Potassium Banana Bread

Day 11:

- Breakfast: Chia Seed Pudding
- Lunch: Turkey and Avocado Wrap
- Dinner: Spinach and Goat Cheese Stuffed Chicken
- Snacks: Caprese Skewers
- Dessert: Greek Yogurt with Honey

Day 12:

- Breakfast: Cottage Cheese and Fruit
- Lunch: Zucchini Noodles with Pesto
- Dinner: Low-Potassium Chili

- Snacks: Mini Quiches with Kidney-Friendly Fillings
- Dessert: Almond Butter Cookies (in moderation)

Day 13:

- Breakfast: Breakfast Quiche with Low-Potassium Veggies
- Lunch: BBQ Chicken Skewers
- Dinner: Roasted Vegetable Lasagna
- Snacks: Greek Tzatziki with Pita
- Dessert: Baked Apples

Day 14:

- Breakfast: Buckwheat Pancakes
- Lunch: Egg Salad Lettuce Wraps
- Dinner: Lemon Garlic Tilapia
- Snacks: Stuffed Mushrooms
- Dessert: Strawberry Shortcake

Week 3:

Day 15:

- Breakfast: Oatmeal Cookies (in moderation)
- Lunch: Cauliflower Rice Bowl

- Dinner: Ratatouille
- Snacks: Low-Potassium Bruschetta
- Dessert: Peach Cobbler (in moderation)

Day 16:

- Breakfast: Rice Cake with Almond Butter
- Lunch: Beef and Vegetable Stew
- Dinner: Creamy Potato Soup
- Snacks: Antipasto Platter
- Dessert: Coconut Rice Pudding

Day 17:

- Breakfast: Breakfast Tacos
- Lunch: Caprese Salad
- Dinner: Vegetarian Tikka Masala
- Snacks: Spinach and Artichoke Dip
- Dessert: Carrot Cake (in moderation)

Day 18:

- Breakfast: Veggie Scramble
- Lunch: Asian-style Tofu Bowl
- Dinner: Spaghetti Squash with Pesto

- Snacks: Deviled Eggs (in moderation)
- Dessert: Baked Apples

Day 19:

- Breakfast: Low-Potassium Oatmeal with Berries
- Lunch: Chicken and Vegetable Stir-Fry
- Dinner: Grilled Chicken Breast with Lemon
- Snacks: Veggie Sticks with Hummus
- Dessert: Berry Parfait with Whipped Cream

Day 20:

- Breakfast: Scrambled Egg Whites with Spinach
- Lunch: Tuna Salad with Low-Potassium Ingredients
- Dinner: Baked Cod with Herbed Potatoes
- Snacks: Low-Potassium Salsa and Chips
- Dessert: Apple Crisp (in moderation)

Day 21:

- Breakfast: Greek Yogurt Parfait with Nuts
- Lunch: Quinoa and Chickpea Salad
- Dinner: Quinoa-Stuffed Bell Peppers
- Snacks: Cottage Cheese Dip with Veggies

- Dessert: Chocolate Avocado Mousse

Week 4

Day 22:

- Breakfast: Banana-Free Smoothie
- Lunch: Turkey Wrap with Hummus
- Dinner: Beef and Broccoli Stir-Fry
- Snacks: Guacamole with Cucumber Slices
- Dessert: Poached Pears

Day 23:

- Breakfast: Quinoa Breakfast Bowl
- Lunch: Baked Salmon with Herbs
- Dinner: Eggplant Parmesan
- Snacks: Roasted Chickpeas
- Dessert: Rice Pudding (in moderation)

Day 24:

- Breakfast: Avocado Toast with Low-Potassium Toppings
- Lunch: Spinach and Lentil Soup
- Dinner: Teriyaki Salmon

- Snacks: Mixed Nuts (in moderation)
- Dessert: Angel Food Cake with Berries

Day 25:

- Breakfast: Cereal Alternatives
- Lunch: Low-Potassium Pasta Salad
- Dinner: Creamy Mushroom Risotto
- Snacks: Fruit Sorbet
- Dessert: Lemon Sorbet

Day 26:

- Breakfast: Sweet Potato Hash Browns
- Lunch: Lentil and Vegetable Curry
- Dinner: Lemon Herb Shrimp
- Snacks: Rice Cakes with Toppings
- Dessert: Pumpkin Pie (in moderation)

Day 27:

- Breakfast: Low-Potassium Pancakes
- Lunch: Greek Salad with Feta
- Dinner: Stuffed Cabbage Rolls
- Snacks: Baked Sweet Potato Fries

- Dessert: Chia Seed Chocolate Pudding

Day 28:

- Breakfast: Breakfast Burrito with Kidney-Friendly Ingredients
- Lunch: Roasted Veggie and Couscous Bowl
- Dinner: Pork Tenderloin with Apple Sauce
- Snacks: Edamame
- Dessert: Low-Potassium Banana Bread

Day 29:

- Breakfast: Chia Seed Pudding
- Lunch: Turkey and Avocado Wrap
- Dinner: Spinach and Goat Cheese Stuffed Chicken
- Snacks: Caprese Skewers
- Dessert: Greek Yogurt with Honey

Day 30:

- Breakfast: Cottage Cheese and Fruit
- Lunch: Zucchini Noodles with Pesto
- Dinner: Low-Potassium Chili
- Snacks: Mini Quiches with Kidney-Friendly Fillings

- Dessert: Almond Butter Cookies (in moderation)

Congratulations on completing your 30-day low-potassium meal plan! This diverse and nutritious plan should help support your kidney health while keeping your meals exciting and flavorful.

Chapter 2: Breakfast Recipes

In Chapter 2, we dive into a delightful selection of breakfast recipes specially crafted to support your kidney health by keeping potassium levels in check. These breakfasts are not only delicious but also nourishing, ensuring a great start to your day. Let's explore these morning delights together.

Low-Potassium Oatmeal with Berries

Ingredients:

- 1/2 cup rolled oats
- 1/2 cup almond milk
- 1/4 cup fresh mixed berries
- 1 tablespoon honey
- 1/4 teaspoon cinnamon

Instructions:

1. Combine oats and almond milk in a saucepan.
2. Cook over medium heat until creamy, stirring occasionally.

3. Top with fresh berries, honey, and a sprinkle of cinnamon.

Scrambled Egg Whites with Spinach

Ingredients:

- 3 egg whites
- 1/2 cup fresh spinach leaves
- Salt and pepper to taste
- Cooking spray

Instructions:

1. Whisk egg whites with salt and pepper.
2. Heat a non-stick pan and coat with cooking spray.
3. Add spinach and pour in the egg whites.
4. Cook, stirring gently until eggs are set.

Greek Yogurt Parfait with Nuts

Ingredients:

- 1/2 cup Greek yogurt
- 1/4 cup chopped mixed nuts (almonds, walnuts)
- 1/4 cup fresh berries

- 1 tablespoon honey

Instructions:

1. Layer Greek yogurt, nuts, and berries in a glass.
2. Drizzle honey over the top.
3. Enjoy this protein-packed parfait.

Banana-Free Smoothie

Ingredients:

- 1 cup unsweetened almond milk
- 1/2 cup frozen mixed berries
- 1/4 cup spinach
- 1 tablespoon chia seeds
- 1 teaspoon honey (optional)

Instructions:

1. Blend almond milk, berries, spinach, and chia seeds until smooth.
2. Add honey for sweetness if desired.
3. Sip on this potassium-friendly smoothie.

Quinoa Breakfast Bowl

Ingredients:

- 1/2 cup cooked quinoa
- 1/4 cup sliced strawberries
- 1/4 cup chopped almonds
- 1/4 teaspoon vanilla extract

Instructions:

1. Mix cooked quinoa with vanilla extract.
2. Top with strawberries and chopped almonds.
3. A nutritious and hearty start to your day.

Avocado Toast with Low-Potassium Toppings

Ingredients:

- 1 slice whole-grain bread
- 1/4 ripe avocado, mashed
- Sliced cucumber
- Cherry tomatoes, halved
- Sprinkle of sesame seeds

Instructions:

1. Spread mashed avocado on toasted bread.
2. Top with cucumber slices, cherry tomatoes, and sesame seeds.

Cereal Alternatives

Ingredients:

- Choose a low-potassium cereal of your choice.
- Substitute regular milk with almond or rice milk.

Instructions:

1. Pour cereal into a bowl.
2. Add your choice of non-dairy milk.
3. Enjoy a quick and easy breakfast.

Spinach and Feta Omelette

Ingredients:

- 2 egg whites
- Handful of fresh spinach
- 1 tablespoon crumbled feta cheese
- Salt and pepper to taste

Instructions:

1. Whisk egg whites with salt and pepper.

2. Pour into a heated pan.

3. Add spinach and feta, fold in half, and cook until set.

Sweet Potato Hash Browns

Ingredients:

- 1 medium sweet potato, grated

- 1/4 teaspoon paprika

- Salt and pepper to taste

- Cooking spray

Instructions:

1. Toss grated sweet potato with paprika, salt, and pepper.

2. Heat a pan with cooking spray.

3. Cook the sweet potato until crispy and golden brown.

Low-Potassium Pancakes

Ingredients:

- 1/2 cup oat flour

- 1/2 cup unsweetened almond milk
- 1/4 cup unsweetened applesauce
- 1/4 teaspoon baking powder
- Dash of cinnamon

Instructions:

1. Mix oat flour, almond milk, applesauce, baking powder, and cinnamon.
2. Heat a non-stick pan and pour batter to make pancakes.

Breakfast Burrito with Kidney-Friendly Ingredients

Ingredients:

- 1 whole-grain tortilla
- 2 egg whites
- Salsa (low-potassium)
- Sliced avocado
- Chopped cilantro (optional)

Instructions:

1. Scramble egg whites and place on the tortilla.

2. Add salsa, sliced avocado, and cilantro if desired.

3. Roll it up for a satisfying breakfast.

Chia Seed Pudding

Ingredients:

- 2 tablespoons chia seeds

- 1/2 cup unsweetened almond milk

- 1/4 teaspoon vanilla extract

- Sliced strawberries (optional)

Instructions:

1. Mix chia seeds, almond milk, and vanilla extract.

2. Refrigerate overnight or for a few hours.

3. Top with sliced strawberries before serving.

Cottage Cheese and Fruit

Ingredients:

- 1/2 cup low-fat cottage cheese

- Sliced peaches or pears (low-potassium)

Instructions:

1. Serve a scoop of cottage cheese with sliced peaches
    or pears.

2. A simple and protein-rich breakfast.

Breakfast Quiche with Low-Potassium Veggies

Ingredients:

- 2 egg whites
- Chopped low-potassium veggies (e.g., bell peppers, zucchini)
- 1 tablespoon shredded low-fat cheese (optional)
- Salt and pepper to taste

Instructions:

1. Whisk egg whites and pour into a greased muffin tin.
2. Add chopped veggies and cheese if desired.
3. Bake until quiches are set.

Buckwheat Pancakes

Ingredients:

- 1/2 cup buckwheat flour
- 1/2 cup almond milk
- 1/4 teaspoon baking powder
- Dash of honey (optional)

Instructions:

1. Mix buckwheat flour, almond milk, baking powder, and honey (if desired).
2. Cook pancakes on a griddle until golden.

Rice Cake with Almond Butter

Ingredients:

- 1 rice cake
- 1 tablespoon almond butter (low-potassium)

Instructions:

1. Spread almond butter on a rice cake.
2. A quick and crunchy breakfast option.

Breakfast Tacos

Ingredients:

- 2 small corn tortillas
- Scrambled egg whites
- Salsa (low-potassium)
- Sliced avocado

Instructions:

1. Fill tortillas with scrambled egg whites, salsa, and avocado slices.
2. Roll up for a tasty breakfast taco.

Veggie Scramble

Ingredients:

- 2 egg whites
- Chopped low-potassium veggies (e.g., spinach, bell peppers)
- Sliced mushrooms
- Salt and pepper to taste

Instructions:

1. Scramble egg whites in a pan.

2. Add chopped veggies and mushrooms.

3. Season with salt and pepper.

Chapter 3: Lunch Recipes

In this chapter, we've curated delicious lunch recipes tailored to support kidney health. Each recipe is thoughtfully crafted to be low in potassium, ensuring that you can enjoy a satisfying meal without compromising your dietary needs. Let's dive into these flavorful and kidney-friendly lunch options:

Chicken and Vegetable Stir-Fry

Ingredients:

- 2 boneless, skinless chicken breasts
- Assorted vegetables (bell peppers, broccoli, carrots)
- Low-sodium stir-fry sauce
- Olive oil
- Cooked quinoa (optional)

Instructions:

1. Cut chicken into bite-sized pieces and stir-fry until cooked.
2. Add assorted vegetables and stir-fry until tender.

3. Drizzle with low-sodium stir-fry sauce.

4. Serve over cooked quinoa if desired.

Tuna Salad with Low-Potassium Ingredients

Ingredients:

- Canned tuna in water
- Chopped celery
- Chopped red onion
- Greek yogurt (as a mayo substitute)
- Lemon juice
- Salt and pepper to taste
- Lettuce leaves

Instructions:

1. Mix tuna, celery, red onion, and Greek yogurt.

2. Add lemon juice, salt, and pepper to taste.

3. Serve in lettuce leaves for a fresh wrap.

Quinoa and Chickpea Salad

Ingredients:

- Cooked quinoa
- Cooked chickpeas
- Diced cucumber
- Chopped fresh parsley
- Lemon vinaigrette dressing
- Feta cheese (optional)

Instructions:

1. Combine quinoa, chickpeas, cucumber, and parsley.
2. Drizzle with lemon vinaigrette dressing.
3. Add crumbled feta cheese if desired.

Turkey Wrap with Hummus

Ingredients:

- Sliced turkey breast
- Whole-grain tortilla
- Hummus
- Sliced cucumber and tomato
- Lettuce leaves

Instructions:
1. Spread hummus on the tortilla.
2. Layer turkey, cucumber, tomato, and lettuce.
3. Roll up and enjoy.

Baked Salmon with Herbs

Ingredients:
- Salmon fillet
- Fresh herbs (rosemary, thyme)
- Lemon slices
- Olive oil
- Salt and pepper

Instructions:
1. Place salmon on a baking sheet.
2. Top with fresh herbs, lemon slices, olive oil, salt, and pepper.
3. Bake until salmon flakes easily.

Spinach and Lentil Soup

Ingredients:

- Lentils
- Chopped spinach
- Low-sodium vegetable broth
- Chopped onion and garlic
- Olive oil
- Spices (cumin, coriander)

Instructions:

1. Sauté onion and garlic in olive oil.
2. Add lentils, spinach, vegetable broth, and spices.
3. Simmer until lentils are tender.

Low-Potassium Pasta Salad

Ingredients:

- Whole-grain pasta
- Cherry tomatoes
- Cucumber
- Red onion
- Italian dressing

- Fresh basil

Instructions:

1. Cook pasta and cool.
2. Mix with chopped tomatoes, cucumber, red onion, Italian dressing, and fresh basil.

Lentil and Vegetable Curry

Ingredients:

- Red lentils
- Assorted vegetables (bell peppers, carrots, peas)
- Curry paste
- Coconut milk
- Fresh cilantro

Instructions:

1. Cook red lentils until soft.
2. Sauté vegetables in curry paste.
3. Add cooked lentils and coconut milk.
4. Simmer until vegetables are tender.
5. Garnish with fresh cilantro.

Greek Salad with Feta

Ingredients:

- Cucumber
- Cherry tomatoes
- Red onion
- Kalamata olives
- Feta cheese
- Greek dressing
- Fresh oregano

Instructions:

1. Chop cucumber, tomatoes, red onion, and olives.
2. Toss with crumbled feta cheese and Greek dressing.
3. Sprinkle with fresh oregano.

Roasted Veggie and Couscous Bowl

Ingredients:

- Assorted roasted vegetables (zucchini, bell peppers, eggplant)
- Cooked couscous
- Balsamic vinaigrette

- Fresh basil

Instructions:

1. Roast vegetables until tender.

2. Serve over cooked couscous.

3. Drizzle with balsamic vinaigrette and top with fresh basil.

Turkey and Avocado Wrap

Ingredients:

- Sliced turkey breast
- Avocado slices
- Whole-grain wrap
- Lettuce leaves
- Dijon mustard

Instructions:

1. Spread Dijon mustard on the wrap.

2. Layer turkey, avocado, and lettuce.

3. Roll up for a satisfying wrap.

Zucchini Noodles with Pesto

Ingredients:

- Zucchini noodles
- Homemade or store-bought pesto sauce
- Cherry tomatoes
- Grated Parmesan cheese (optional)

Instructions:

1. Toss zucchini noodles with pesto sauce.
2. Add halved cherry tomatoes.
3. Sprinkle with grated Parmesan cheese if desired.

BBQ Chicken Skewers

Ingredients:

- Chicken breast chunks
- Low-potassium BBQ sauce
- Bell peppers and onions (for skewers)

Instructions:

1. Marinate chicken in low-potassium BBQ sauce.
2. Thread onto skewers with bell peppers and onions.

3. Grill until chicken is cooked through.

Egg Salad Lettuce Wraps

Ingredients:

- Hard-boiled eggs
- Greek yogurt (as a mayo substitute)
- Diced celery and green onion
- Lettuce leaves

Instructions:

1. Mix chopped eggs, Greek yogurt, celery, and green onion.
2. Serve in lettuce leaves for a carb-conscious wrap.

Cauliflower Rice Bowl

Ingredients:

- Cauliflower rice
- Sautéed vegetables
- Grilled chicken or tofu
- Teriyaki sauce (low-potassium)

Instructions:

1. Sauté cauliflower rice and vegetables.
2. Top with grilled chicken or tofu.
3. Drizzle with low-potassium teriyaki sauce.

Beef and Vegetable Stew

Ingredients:

- Lean beef chunks
- Assorted vegetables (carrots, potatoes, green beans)
- Low-sodium beef broth
- Herbs and spices (thyme, rosemary)
- Olive oil

Instructions:

1. Sear beef in olive oil until browned.
2. Add vegetables, broth, and herbs.
3. Simmer until beef is tender.

Caprese Salad

Ingredients:

- Tomato slices

- Fresh mozzarella slices
- Fresh basil leaves
- Balsamic glaze
- Olive oil
- Salt and pepper

Instructions:

1. Layer tomato, mozzarella, and basil.
2. Drizzle with balsamic glaze and olive oil.
3. Season with salt and pepper.

Asian-style Tofu Bowl

Ingredients:

- Tofu cubes
- Stir-fry vegetables
- Low-sodium soy sauce
- Sesame oil
- Steamed rice (optional)

Instructions:

1. Sauté tofu and stir-fry vegetables.
2. Add low-sodium soy sauce and sesame oil.

3.   Serve over steamed rice if desired.

Chapter 4: Dinner Recipes

In this chapter, we explore a delightful array of dinner recipes designed to satisfy your taste buds while adhering to a low-potassium diet. From succulent meats to flavorful vegetarian options, you'll discover a diverse range of dishes that make dinner time a joy. Let's dive into these wholesome recipes.

Grilled Chicken Breast with Lemon

Ingredients:

- 4 boneless, skinless chicken breasts
- 2 lemons, juiced and zested
- 2 cloves garlic, minced
- 2 tablespoons olive oil
- Salt and pepper to taste

Instructions:

1. In a bowl, mix lemon juice, lemon zest, minced garlic, olive oil, salt, and pepper.

2. Marinate chicken breasts in the mixture for at least 30 minutes.

3. Preheat grill to medium-high heat and grill chicken for about 6-8 minutes per side, or until cooked through.

4. Serve with a drizzle of fresh lemon juice.

Baked Cod with Herbed Potatoes

Ingredients:

- 4 cod fillets
- 4 large potatoes, peeled and sliced
- 2 tablespoons olive oil
- 1 teaspoon dried thyme
- 1 teaspoon dried rosemary
- Salt and pepper to taste

Instructions:

1. Preheat oven to 375°F (190°C).

2. Place cod fillets and sliced potatoes in a baking dish.

3. Drizzle with olive oil and sprinkle with thyme, rosemary, salt, and pepper.

4. Cover with foil and bake for 25-30 minutes, or until the fish flakes easily with a fork.

5. Serve hot.

Quinoa-Stuffed Bell Peppers

Ingredients:

- 4 bell peppers, any color
- 1 cup quinoa, cooked
- 1 cup black beans, drained and rinsed
- 1 cup diced tomatoes
- 1/2 cup corn kernels
- 1/2 cup diced onion
- 1 teaspoon chili powder
- 1/2 teaspoon cumin
- Salt and pepper to taste

Instructions:

1. Preheat oven to 375°F (190°C).

2. Cut the tops off the bell peppers and remove seeds.

3. In a bowl, mix cooked quinoa, black beans, diced tomatoes, corn, diced onion, chili powder, cumin, salt, and pepper.

4. Stuff the bell peppers with the quinoa mixture.

5. Place the stuffed peppers in a baking dish, cover with foil, and bake for 25-30 minutes.

6. Serve hot.

Beef and Broccoli Stir-Fry

Ingredients:

- 1 pound lean beef, thinly sliced
- 2 cups broccoli florets
- 1/4 cup low-sodium soy sauce
- 2 cloves garlic, minced
- 1 tablespoon ginger, minced
- 2 tablespoons vegetable oil
- 1 tablespoon cornstarch
- 2 tablespoons water

Instructions:

1. In a small bowl, whisk together soy sauce, minced garlic, minced ginger, cornstarch, and water.

2. Heat vegetable oil in a pan over medium-high heat.

3. Add sliced beef and stir-fry until browned.

4. Add broccoli and continue to stir-fry for a few minutes.

5. Pour the soy sauce mixture over the beef and broccoli, stirring until the sauce thickens.

6. Serve hot over rice or noodles.

Eggplant Parmesan

Ingredients:

- 2 large eggplants, sliced into rounds
- 2 cups marinara sauce (low-potassium)
- 2 cups mozzarella cheese, shredded
- 1/2 cup Parmesan cheese, grated
- 1/2 cup breadcrumbs
- 2 tablespoons olive oil
- Salt and pepper to taste
- Fresh basil leaves for garnish

Instructions:

1. Preheat your oven to 375°F (190°C).

2. Dip eggplant slices in egg, then coat with breadcrumbs.

3. Heat olive oil in a pan over medium heat and fry eggplant slices until golden brown.

4. In a baking dish, spread a layer of marinara sauce, followed by a layer of eggplant slices, and a layer of mozzarella and Parmesan cheese. Repeat.

5. Bake for 25-30 minutes, or until the cheese is bubbly and golden.

6. Garnish with fresh basil leaves and serve.

Teriyaki Salmon

Ingredients:

- 4 salmon fillets
- 1/4 cup low-sodium teriyaki sauce
- 2 tablespoons honey
- 1 tablespoon minced ginger
- 2 cloves garlic, minced
- Sesame seeds for garnish
- Sliced green onions for garnish

Instructions:

1. In a bowl, whisk together teriyaki sauce, honey, minced ginger, and minced garlic.

2. Marinate salmon fillets in the mixture for at least 30 minutes.

3. Preheat grill or pan to medium-high heat.

4. Grill or pan-sear salmon for about 4-5 minutes per side, or until cooked to your liking.

5. Garnish with sesame seeds and sliced green onions.

Creamy Mushroom Risotto

Ingredients:

- 1 cup Arborio rice
- 2 cups low-sodium vegetable broth
- 2 cups mushrooms, sliced
- 1/2 cup diced onion
- 2 cloves garlic, minced
- 1/2 cup white wine (optional)
- 2 tablespoons olive oil
- 1/4 cup Parmesan cheese, grated
- Salt and pepper to taste
- Fresh parsley for garnish

Instructions:

1. In a saucepan, heat olive oil over medium heat. Add diced onion and garlic and sauté until softened.

2. Add Arborio rice and cook, stirring, for a few minutes until it becomes translucent.

3. Pour in white wine (if using) and cook until it's mostly absorbed.

4. Gradually add vegetable broth, one ladle at a time, stirring continuously until absorbed before adding more.

5. Stir in sliced mushrooms and continue to cook until rice is creamy and tender.

6. Stir in Parmesan cheese, salt, and pepper.

7. Garnish with fresh parsley and serve.

Lemon Herb Shrimp

Ingredients:

- 1 pound large shrimp, peeled and deveined
- 2 tablespoons olive oil
- 2 cloves garlic, minced
- 1 lemon, juiced and zested
- 1 tablespoon fresh basil, chopped

- 1 tablespoon fresh parsley, chopped
- Salt and pepper to taste

Instructions:

1. In a bowl, combine olive oil, minced garlic, lemon juice, lemon zest, fresh basil, fresh parsley, salt, and pepper.
2. Add shrimp to the mixture and let them marinate for 15-20 minutes.
3. Heat a skillet over medium-high heat and add the marinated shrimp.
4. Cook for about 2-3 minutes per side until they turn pink and opaque.
5. Serve hot, garnished with extra herbs and lemon slices.

Stuffed Cabbage Rolls

Ingredients:

- 1 large cabbage
- 1 pound ground beef or turkey
- 1 cup cooked rice
- 1/2 cup diced onion

- 1 can low-sodium tomato sauce

- 2 cloves garlic, minced

- Salt and pepper to taste

Instructions:

1. Carefully remove the cabbage leaves and blanch them in boiling water for a few minutes until soft.

2. In a bowl, combine ground meat, cooked rice, diced onion, minced garlic, salt, and pepper.

3. Place a spoonful of the meat mixture in the center of each cabbage leaf and roll them up.

4. Place the cabbage rolls in a baking dish and pour tomato sauce over them.

5. Cover with foil and bake at 350°F (175°C) for about 45 minutes to an hour.

6. Serve with additional tomato sauce if desired.

Pork Tenderloin with Apple Sauce

Ingredients:

- 1 pork tenderloin

- 2 apples, peeled, cored, and sliced

- 1/4 cup unsweetened applesauce

- 1/4 cup low-sodium chicken broth
- 1 tablespoon honey
- 1 teaspoon cinnamon
- Salt and pepper to taste

Instructions:

1. Season pork tenderloin with salt and pepper.
2. In a skillet, sear the pork on all sides until browned.
3. In a separate saucepan, combine apples, applesauce, chicken broth, honey, and cinnamon.
4. Simmer until apples are soft and sauce is thickened.
5. Slice the pork tenderloin and serve with apple sauce.

Spinach and Goat Cheese Stuffed Chicken

Ingredients:

- 4 boneless, skinless chicken breasts
- 1 cup fresh spinach leaves
- 1/2 cup goat cheese, crumbled
- 2 cloves garlic, minced
- Salt and pepper to taste

- Olive oil for cooking

Instructions:

1. Preheat your oven to 375°F (190°C).
2. Cut a pocket into each chicken breast.
3. In a bowl, mix together fresh spinach, goat cheese, minced garlic, salt, and pepper.
4. Stuff each chicken breast with the spinach and goat cheese mixture.
5. Heat olive oil in an oven-safe skillet over medium-high heat.
6. Sear chicken breasts for about 2-3 minutes per side until they develop a golden crust.
7. Transfer the skillet to the preheated oven and bake for 15-20 minutes, or until the chicken is cooked through.
8. Serve hot.

Low-Potassium Chili

Ingredients:

- 1 pound ground turkey
- 1 can low-sodium kidney beans, drained and rinsed

- 1 can low-sodium black beans, drained and rinsed
- 1 can low-sodium diced tomatoes
- 1/2 cup diced onion
- 2 cloves garlic, minced
- 1 tablespoon chili powder
- 1 teaspoon cumin
- Salt and pepper to taste

Instructions:

1. In a large pot, cook ground turkey over medium heat until browned.
2. Add diced onion and minced garlic, cooking until they soften.
3. Stir in kidney beans, black beans, diced tomatoes, chili powder, cumin, salt, and pepper.
4. Simmer for 20-30 minutes, allowing flavors to meld.
5. Serve with low-potassium toppings like chopped green onions or a dollop of low-potassium sour cream.

Roasted Vegetable Lasagna

Ingredients:

- 9 lasagna noodles, cooked
- 2 cups ricotta cheese (low-sodium)
- 2 cups mozzarella cheese, shredded
- 2 cups roasted mixed vegetables (zucchini, bell peppers, eggplant, etc.)
- 2 cups low-sodium marinara sauce
- 1/4 cup Parmesan cheese, grated
- Salt and pepper to taste

Instructions:

1. Preheat your oven to 375°F (190°C).
2. In a bowl, mix together ricotta cheese, half of the mozzarella cheese, salt, and pepper.
3. In a baking dish, layer cooked lasagna noodles, roasted vegetables, ricotta mixture, and marinara sauce.
4. Repeat the layers until all ingredients are used.
5. Top with the remaining mozzarella and Parmesan cheese.

6. Cover with foil and bake for 25-30 minutes, then uncover and bake for an additional 10-15 minutes until cheese is bubbly and golden.

7. Let it cool slightly before serving.

Lemon Garlic Tilapia

Ingredients:

- 4 tilapia fillets
- 2 lemons, juiced and zested
- 4 cloves garlic, minced
- 2 tablespoons olive oil
- Salt and pepper to taste
- Fresh parsley for garnish

Instructions:

1. In a bowl, combine lemon juice, lemon zest, minced garlic, olive oil, salt, and pepper.

2. Marinate tilapia fillets in the mixture for at least 15 minutes.

3. Heat a skillet over medium-high heat and cook tilapia for about 3-4 minutes per side until it flakes easily.

4. Garnish with fresh parsley and serve.

Ratatouille

Ingredients:

- 2 zucchinis, sliced
- 1 eggplant, cubed
- 2 red bell peppers, sliced
- 1 onion, chopped
- 2 cloves garlic, minced
- 2 cups diced tomatoes (low-sodium)
- 2 tablespoons olive oil
- 1 teaspoon dried thyme
- 1 teaspoon dried basil
- Salt and pepper to taste
- Fresh basil leaves for garnish

Instructions:

1. Heat olive oil in a large skillet over medium heat.
2. Add chopped onion and minced garlic, sauté until softened.
3. Add zucchini, eggplant, red bell peppers, dried thyme, dried basil, salt, and pepper.
4. Cook, stirring occasionally, for about 10 minutes until vegetables are tender.

5. Stir in diced tomatoes and simmer for an additional
    5 minutes.

6. Garnish with fresh basil leaves and serve.

Creamy Potato Soup

Ingredients:

- 4 large potatoes, peeled and diced
- 1 onion, chopped
- 2 cloves garlic, minced
- 4 cups low-sodium vegetable broth
- 1 cup low-fat milk
- 2 tablespoons butter (or butter substitute)
- Salt and pepper to taste
- Chopped chives for garnish

Instructions:

1. In a large pot, melt butter over medium heat.

2. Add chopped onion and minced garlic, sauté until
    translucent.

3. Add diced potatoes and vegetable broth, bring to a
    boil, then reduce heat and simmer until potatoes are
    tender.

4. Use an immersion blender to puree the soup until smooth.

5. Stir in low-fat milk and heat through.

6. Season with salt and pepper.

7. Garnish with chopped chives and serve.

Vegetarian Tikka Masala

Ingredients:

- 2 cups cauliflower florets
- 2 cups chickpeas, cooked
- 1 cup low-fat yogurt
- 1 onion, chopped
- 2 cloves garlic, minced
- 2 teaspoons curry powder
- 1 teaspoon garam masala
- 1 teaspoon turmeric
- Salt and pepper to taste
- Fresh cilantro leaves for garnish

Instructions:

1. In a large skillet, heat olive oil over medium heat.

2. Add chopped onion and minced garlic, sauté until softened.

3. Stir in curry powder, garam masala, turmeric, salt, and pepper.

4. Add cauliflower florets and chickpeas, cooking for a few minutes.

5. Pour in low-fat yogurt and simmer until the sauce thickens.

6. Garnish with fresh cilantro leaves and serve over rice or with naan bread.

Spaghetti Squash with Pesto

Ingredients:

- 1 spaghetti squash, halved and seeds removed
- 1 cup basil leaves
- 1/4 cup pine nuts
- 1/4 cup grated Parmesan cheese
- 2 cloves garlic, minced
- 1/4 cup olive oil
- Salt and pepper to taste

Instructions:

1. Preheat your oven to 375°F (190°C).

2. Place spaghetti squash halves cut side down on a baking sheet and roast for about 45 minutes, or until the flesh is tender.

3. While the squash is roasting, prepare the pesto by blending basil leaves, pine nuts, grated Parmesan cheese, minced garlic, olive oil, salt, and pepper in a food processor.

4. Use a fork to scrape the spaghetti-like strands of the cooked squash.

5. Toss the squash with the prepared pesto.

6. Serve as a flavorful, low-potassium pasta alternative.

Chapter 5: Snacks and Appetizers

In this chapter, we've curated a diverse selection of snacks and appetizers that are not only low in potassium but also bursting with flavor. From crunchy veggie sticks with creamy hummus to zesty low-potassium salsa with chips, you'll discover a range of options to please your palate.

Veggie Sticks with Hummus

Ingredients:

- Assorted fresh vegetables (carrots, cucumbers, bell peppers)
- Hummus

Instructions:

1. Wash and cut the vegetables into sticks.
2. Serve them with a generous portion of hummus for dipping.

Low-Potassium Salsa and Chips

Ingredients:

- Low-potassium salsa (homemade or store-bought)
- Low-sodium tortilla chips

Instructions:

1. Pour the salsa into a serving bowl.
2. Arrange tortilla chips on a platter.
3. Dip and enjoy!

Cottage Cheese Dip with Veggies

Ingredients:

- Low-fat cottage cheese
- Assorted fresh vegetables for dipping (celery, cherry tomatoes, cucumber)

Instructions:

1. Spoon cottage cheese into a bowl.
2. Wash and chop the veggies.
3. Dip and savor the combination of textures and flavors.

Guacamole with Cucumber Slices

Ingredients:

- Ripe avocados
- Lime juice
- Onion
- Tomato
- Garlic
- Cilantro
- Cucumber slices

Instructions:

1. Mash the avocados and mix with lime juice.
2. Add finely chopped onion, tomato, garlic, and cilantro.
3. Serve with crisp cucumber slices.

Roasted Chickpeas

Ingredients:

- Canned chickpeas (rinsed and drained)
- Olive oil
- Seasonings (paprika, cumin, garlic powder)

- Salt

Instructions:

1. Toss chickpeas with olive oil and seasonings.
2. Roast in the oven until crispy.
3. Sprinkle with a pinch of salt and enjoy the crunch!

Mixed Nuts (in moderation)

Ingredients:

- Assorted unsalted nuts (almonds, walnuts, pistachios)

Instructions:

1. Portion a small mix of nuts for a satisfying snack.
2. Remember to consume in moderation due to potassium content.

Fruit Sorbet

Ingredients:

- Frozen low-potassium fruits (like berries or peaches)
- Sweetener (optional)

Instructions:

1. Blend the frozen fruits until smooth.

2. Add sweetener if desired.

3. Scoop and serve this refreshing sorbet.

Rice Cakes with Toppings

Ingredients:

- Low-potassium rice cakes
- Toppings (hummus, sliced cucumber, cherry tomatoes)

Instructions:

1. Top rice cakes with a dollop of hummus, cucumber slices, and cherry tomatoes.

2. Create your own combinations for variety.

Baked Sweet Potato Fries

Ingredients:

- Sweet potatoes
- Olive oil
- Seasonings (paprika, garlic powder, salt)

Instructions:

1. Cut sweet potatoes into fries.
2. Toss with olive oil and seasonings.
3. Bake until crispy and delicious.

Edamame

Ingredients:

- Edamame pods
- Salt

Instructions:

1. Steam or boil edamame until tender.
2. Sprinkle with a pinch of salt and enjoy these protein-packed green gems.

Caprese Skewers

Ingredients:

- Cherry tomatoes
- Fresh basil leaves
- Mozzarella cheese balls
- Balsamic glaze (optional)

Instructions:

1. Thread cherry tomatoes, fresh basil leaves, and mozzarella cheese balls onto skewers.
2. Drizzle with balsamic glaze if desired for a burst of flavor.

Mini Quiches with Kidney-Friendly Fillings

Ingredients:

- Mini quiche shells (store-bought or homemade)
- Low-potassium fillings (spinach, mushrooms, low-potassium cheese)
- Eggs
- Milk (or milk substitute)
- Seasonings

Instructions:

1. Preheat the oven and prepare quiche shells.
2. Fill with kidney-friendly ingredients.
3. Whisk eggs, milk, and seasonings together, then pour into the shells.

4. Bake until set and golden.

Greek Tzatziki with Pita

Ingredients:

- Greek yogurt
- Cucumber
- Garlic
- Lemon juice
- Fresh dill
- Whole wheat pita bread

Instructions:

1. Grate cucumber and squeeze out excess moisture.
2. Mix with Greek yogurt, minced garlic, lemon juice, and fresh dill to make tzatziki.
3. Serve with toasted pita bread.

Stuffed Mushrooms

Ingredients:

- Fresh mushrooms

- Low-potassium stuffing (breadcrumbs, herbs, and spices)
- Olive oil

Instructions:

1. Remove mushroom stems and hollow out caps.
2. Fill with a flavorful low-potassium stuffing mixture.
3. Bake until mushrooms are tender and stuffing is golden.

Low-Potassium Bruschetta

Ingredients:

- Whole grain baguette slices
- Tomato
- Basil
- Garlic
- Olive oil

Instructions:

1. Dice tomatoes, chop basil, and mince garlic.
2. Mix with a drizzle of olive oil.

3. Spoon onto toasted baguette slices for a classic bruschetta.

Antipasto Platter

Ingredients:

- Low-potassium deli meats (like turkey)
- Low-potassium cheeses
- Olives
- Roasted red peppers
- Pickles

Instructions:

1. Arrange a variety of antipasto items on a platter for a Mediterranean-inspired feast.

Spinach and Artichoke Dip

Ingredients:

- Spinach
- Artichoke hearts
- Greek yogurt
- Parmesan cheese

- Garlic

- Seasonings

- Whole wheat pita chips (for dipping)

Instructions:

1. Combine chopped spinach, artichoke hearts, Greek yogurt, Parmesan cheese, garlic, and seasonings to create a creamy dip.

2. Serve with whole wheat pita chips.

Deviled Eggs (in moderation)

Ingredients:

- Hard-boiled eggs

- Greek yogurt

- Mustard

- Paprika (for garnish)

Instructions:

1. Halve hard-boiled eggs and remove yolks.

2. Mix yolks with Greek yogurt and mustard.

3. Fill egg white halves with the mixture and sprinkle with paprika.

Chapter 6: Desserts

Indulging in a delightful dessert can be the perfect way to conclude a wholesome meal. Here in Chapter 6, we present a collection of 18 delicious desserts that cater to kidney health while satisfying your sweet cravings. Remember, moderation is key, so enjoy these treats responsibly.

Berry Parfait with Whipped Cream

Ingredients:

- 1 cup of low-potassium berries (e.g., strawberries, blueberries, raspberries)
- 1/2 cup of whipped cream (use a low-potassium alternative)
- 1 tablespoon of honey (optional)

Instructions:

1. Layer the berries in a glass or bowl.
2. Top with a dollop of whipped cream.
3. Drizzle with honey if desired.
4. Repeat the layers.

5. Serve chilled.

Apple Crisp (in moderation)

Ingredients:

- 2 cups of sliced apples (choose lower-potassium varieties)
- 1/2 cup of oats
- 2 tablespoons of melted butter (use a low-potassium substitute)
- 2 tablespoons of brown sugar (or a potassium-friendly sweetener)
- 1/2 teaspoon of cinnamon

Instructions:

1. Preheat your oven to 350°F (175°C).
2. Place sliced apples in a baking dish.
3. In a separate bowl, combine oats, melted butter, brown sugar, and cinnamon.
4. Sprinkle the oat mixture evenly over the apples.
5. Bake for 30 minutes or until the topping is golden and the apples are tender.

Chocolate Avocado Mousse

Ingredients:

- 2 ripe avocados
- 1/2 cup of unsweetened cocoa powder
- 1/4 cup of honey (adjust to taste)
- 1 teaspoon of vanilla extract
- A pinch of salt

Instructions:

1. Blend avocados, cocoa powder, honey, vanilla extract, and salt until smooth.
2. Refrigerate for at least 30 minutes.
3. Serve chilled with a garnish of berries.

Poached Pears

Ingredients:

- 4 ripe pears
- 1 cinnamon stick
- 1/4 cup of honey
- 1 lemon (juiced)

Instructions:

1. Peel the pears, leaving the stems intact.

2. In a saucepan, combine water, honey, cinnamon stick, and lemon juice.

3. Add pears and simmer until tender (about 15-20 minutes).

4. Serve with a drizzle of the poaching liquid.

Rice Pudding (in moderation)

Ingredients:

- 1 cup of cooked white rice
- 2 cups of milk (or a low-potassium alternative)
- 1/4 cup of sugar (or a potassium-friendly sweetener)
- 1/2 teaspoon of vanilla extract
- A pinch of cinnamon

Instructions:

1. Combine rice, milk, sugar, and cinnamon in a saucepan.

2. Cook over low heat, stirring often, until thickened (about 20-25 minutes).

3. Remove from heat, stir in vanilla, and let it cool.

4. Serve warm or chilled.

Angel Food Cake with Berries

Ingredients:

- 1 store-bought angel food cake (look for a low-potassium version)
- 2 cups of mixed berries (e.g., strawberries, blueberries, raspberries)
- Low-potassium whipped cream or yogurt for topping

Instructions:

1. Slice the angel food cake into servings.
2. Top each slice with mixed berries.
3. Add a dollop of low-potassium whipped cream or yogurt.
4. Enjoy this light and airy dessert.

Lemon Sorbet

Ingredients:

- 2 cups of fresh lemon juice
- 1 cup of sugar (or a potassium-friendly sweetener)

- 2 cups of water

Instructions:

1. In a saucepan, dissolve sugar in water over medium heat, stirring until clear.
2. Allow the sugar syrup to cool.
3. Stir in fresh lemon juice.
4. Pour the mixture into an ice cream maker and freeze according to the manufacturer's instructions.
5. Once frozen, scoop and serve for a refreshing treat.

Pumpkin Pie (in moderation)

Ingredients:

- 1 pre-made pie crust (look for a low-potassium option)
- 2 cups of canned pumpkin (low-potassium variety)
- 1/2 cup of sugar (or a potassium-friendly sweetener)
- 1/2 teaspoon of cinnamon
- 1/4 teaspoon of nutmeg
- 1/4 teaspoon of cloves
- 2 eggs
- 1 cup of milk (or a low-potassium alternative)

Instructions:

1. Preheat your oven to 425°F (220°C).

2. In a bowl, mix pumpkin, sugar, cinnamon, nutmeg, cloves, eggs, and milk.

3. Pour the mixture into the pie crust.

4. Bake for 15 minutes, then reduce the oven temperature to 350°F (175°C) and bake for an additional 40-50 minutes or until the center is set.

5. Let it cool before serving.

Chia Seed Chocolate Pudding

Ingredients:

- 1/4 cup of chia seeds
- 1 cup of unsweetened almond milk (or a low-potassium alternative)
- 2 tablespoons of unsweetened cocoa powder
- 2 tablespoons of honey (adjust to taste)
- 1/2 teaspoon of vanilla extract

Instructions:

1. In a bowl, whisk together chia seeds, almond milk, cocoa powder, honey, and vanilla extract.

2. Refrigerate for at least 2 hours or overnight until it thickens.

3. Serve with a sprinkle of cocoa powder or fresh berries.

Low-Potassium Banana Bread

Ingredients:

- 2 ripe bananas (choose lower-potassium varieties)
- 1/2 cup of unsweetened applesauce
- 1/4 cup of sugar (or a potassium-friendly sweetener)
- 1 egg
- 1 1/2 cups of all-purpose flour
- 1 teaspoon of baking soda
- 1/2 teaspoon of salt
- 1/2 teaspoon of cinnamon

Instructions:

1. Preheat your oven to 350°F (175°C).

2. Mash bananas and mix with applesauce, sugar, and egg.

3. In a separate bowl, combine flour, baking soda, salt, and cinnamon.

4. Gradually add the dry ingredients to the banana mixture.

5. Pour the batter into a greased loaf pan.

6. Bake for 60-65 minutes or until a toothpick comes out clean.

7. Let it cool before slicing.

Greek Yogurt with Honey

Ingredients:

- 1 cup of low-potassium Greek yogurt
- 2 tablespoons of honey
- Fresh berries for topping (optional)

Instructions:

1. Spoon Greek yogurt into a bowl.

2. Drizzle honey over the yogurt.

3. Add fresh berries for a burst of flavor if desired.

4. Enjoy this simple and nutritious dessert.

Almond Butter Cookies (in moderation)

Ingredients:

- 1 cup of almond butter (low-potassium variety)
- 1/2 cup of sugar (or a potassium-friendly sweetener)
- 1 egg
- 1/2 teaspoon of baking soda
- 1/2 teaspoon of vanilla extract

Instructions:

1. Preheat your oven to 350°F (175°C).
2. In a bowl, mix almond butter, sugar, egg, baking soda, and vanilla extract.
3. Roll the dough into small balls and place them on a baking sheet.
4. Flatten each ball with a fork.
5. Bake for 10-12 minutes or until they're lightly golden.
6. Allow them to cool before enjoying.

Baked Apples

Ingredients:

- 4 apples (choose lower-potassium varieties)
- 1/4 cup of chopped nuts (in moderation)
- 2 tablespoons of honey
- 1/2 teaspoon of cinnamon

Instructions:

1. Preheat your oven to 375°F (190°C).
2. Core the apples, leaving the bottoms intact.
3. In a bowl, mix chopped nuts, honey, and cinnamon.
4. Stuff each apple with the nut mixture.
5. Place the apples in a baking dish and cover with foil.
6. Bake for 30-40 minutes or until the apples are tender.
7. Serve warm.

Strawberry Shortcake

Ingredients:

- Low-potassium shortcakes (store-bought or homemade)
- 2 cups of fresh strawberries, sliced

- Low-potassium whipped cream or yogurt for topping

Instructions:

1. Slice the shortcakes in half horizontally.
2. Layer the bottom half with sliced strawberries.
3. Add a dollop of low-potassium whipped cream or yogurt.
4. Place the top half of the shortcake over it.
5. Garnish with more strawberries.
6. Delight in this classic dessert with a kidney-friendly twist.

Oatmeal Cookies (in moderation)

Ingredients:

- 1 cup of rolled oats
- 1/2 cup of mashed bananas (choose lower-potassium bananas)
- 1/4 cup of unsweetened applesauce
- 1/4 cup of chopped nuts (in moderation)
- 1/4 cup of raisins (in moderation)

Instructions:

1. Preheat your oven to 350°F (175°C).
2. In a bowl, mix rolled oats, mashed bananas, applesauce, nuts, and raisins.
3. Drop spoonfuls of the mixture onto a baking sheet.
4. Flatten each cookie with the back of a fork.
5. Bake for 15-20 minutes or until they're golden.
6. Let them cool before enjoying.

Peach Cobbler (in moderation)

Ingredients:

- 2 cups of sliced peaches (choose lower-potassium varieties)
- 1/2 cup of sugar (or a potassium-friendly sweetener)
- 1 cup of flour
- 1/2 cup of milk (or a low-potassium alternative)
- 1/2 cup of melted butter (use a low-potassium substitute)
- 1 teaspoon of baking powder
- A pinch of salt

Instructions:

1. Preheat your oven to 350°F (175°C).
2. In a baking dish, mix peaches and half of the sugar.
3. In a separate bowl, combine flour, remaining sugar, milk, melted butter, baking powder, and salt.
4. Pour the batter over the peaches.
5. Bake for 30-35 minutes or until the top is golden.
6. Serve warm with a scoop of low-potassium ice cream if desired.

Coconut Rice Pudding

Ingredients:

*   1 cup of cooked rice
*   1 can of coconut milk (low-potassium variety)
*   1/4 cup of sugar (or a potassium-friendly sweetener)
*   1/2 teaspoon of vanilla extract
*   Shredded coconut for garnish

Instructions:

1. In a saucepan, combine cooked rice, coconut milk, sugar, and vanilla extract.

2. Cook over low heat, stirring often, until thickened (about 20-25 minutes).

3. Remove from heat, let it cool, and garnish with shredded coconut.

Carrot Cake (in moderation)

Ingredients:

- 1 cup of grated carrots (choose lower-potassium carrots)
- 1/2 cup of unsweetened applesauce
- 1/4 cup of sugar (or a potassium-friendly sweetener)
- 1/4 cup of vegetable oil (use a low-potassium substitute)
- 1/2 teaspoon of cinnamon
- 1/4 teaspoon of nutmeg
- 1 cup of flour
- 1/2 teaspoon of baking soda
- 1/2 teaspoon of baking powder

Instructions:

1. Preheat your oven to 350°F (175°C).

2. In a bowl, mix grated carrots, applesauce, sugar, vegetable oil, cinnamon, and nutmeg.

3. In another bowl, combine flour, baking soda, and baking powder.

4. Gradually add the dry ingredients to the carrot mixture.

5. Pour the batter into a greased cake pan.

6. Bake for 25-30 minutes or until a toothpick comes out clean.

7. Let it cool before frosting (in moderation).

CONCLUSION

In this final chapter of our journey toward better kidney health through low-potassium meals, we find ourselves at a crossroads, but it's a crossroads filled with newfound knowledge, delicious recipes, and a commitment to wellness.

As we conclude this culinary exploration, it's crucial to reflect on the significance of your efforts. By embarking on this low-potassium dietary path, you've taken a proactive step in preserving and nurturing your kidney health. It's a testament to your dedication to living a vibrant and fulfilling life.

Throughout this book, we've delved into the intricacies of managing potassium intake, creating balanced meal plans, and crafting a diverse array of recipes that are both delectable and kidney-friendly. But the journey doesn't end here; it merely transforms into a lifestyle.

The key takeaway from this chapter is this: consistency is your ally. Sustaining kidney health requires ongoing commitment and mindfulness. Continue to consult with healthcare professionals, monitor your potassium levels, and adapt your meal choices as needed.

Remember, food is not just sustenance; it's a source of joy, connection, and nourishment. Embrace the joy of cooking and sharing meals with loved ones. These moments are more than just opportunities to manage potassium intake; they are occasions to celebrate life's flavors.

As you move forward, explore new ingredients, experiment with recipes, and make this low-potassium lifestyle uniquely yours. Your journey to better kidney health is a testament to your resilience and determination.

In summary, this book is not just about recipes; it's about empowerment. You have the knowledge and tools to make informed choices that positively impact your well-being. Your health is a precious gift, and you are the steward of that gift. May this book be a trusted companion on your continued path to vibrant kidney health.

9 798863 900308